AF887756

X *to* N

The most **POWERFUL** paradigm shift you can make!

J. W. "*JIM*" CAMPBELL

Book 1 "The Story"

We are always interested in finding more stories about things that make us think and the subject of mental fitness. An interactive CD disk to upgrade the quality of your belief system is currently in the works. If you are interested, please email us and you will be placed on the list for the first release.

A cataloguing record for this book includes the U. S. Library of Congress Classification number, the Library of Congress Call number and the Dewey Decimal Cataloguing Code available from the National Library of Congress online database at: http://www.nlc.gov

ISBN: 0-9771647-1-3

This book was published in cooperation with:

J C CAMPBELL PUBLISHING
and
BANNER PRINTING

JC CAMPBELL Publishing,
PO Box 11039 Ft Huachuca, AZ 85670 (503)330-0329
email: jccoregon@hotmail.com

BANNER PRINTING,
342 E. Bartow Dr., Sierra Vista, AZ 85635 (520) 458-5550
email: mackjr@bannerprintingcenter.com

To Jan

MY LIFE'S TRAVELING COMPANION,
CONFIDANT,

AND CRITIC "PAR EXCELLANCE"

CONTENTS

"You're never fully dressed without a smile!"

HOW TO GET THE MOST FROM THIS BOOK

FIRST AND FOREMOST:

Please,.. read "THE STORY" <u>before</u> looking at the check up questions.

SPECIAL NOTICE:

Because the story in this book is about a woman does not mean I am prejudiced against women. It just so happened that the woman in the story was an actual person who came to see me and provided me with the ideal example to use in helping to convert people from X to N. I learned more from her than she did from me.

I am a person – not a plumbing system. Persons are not red, yellow, black or white. Persons are not bodies, but souls or spirits in a body.

THIS BOOK IS INTIMIDATING!

Normally, people are reluctant to answer the check up questions aloud as they are afraid they will give a wrong answer and someone will hear them.

The first time they go through the check up questions they get some of them wrong. I EXPECT them to have mostly incomplete answers and only a few correct answers – the first time through.

The second time through the check up questions they get more correct answers.

The third or fourth time through, they will begin to get them all correct but cannot recite the answers exactly as I have them written. That's OK!

Go through the check up questions until you have enabled yourself to answer every question close to the way it is written in the book. At least understand why I give that answer.

In seminars I require all the students to state the answer to the check up question aloud. Since I'm not with you to ask the questions, I am certain you would get more from the questions if you say your answer aloud before turning the page from the question to the answer.

If you are not in a place where you can answer aloud, try writing at least a synopsis of your answer on a separate piece of paper before turning the page to the answer.

You might give the book to another person and have the person read aloud the check up questions to you. Answer aloud before having him or her read the answer to you. Go through the check up questions at least three to four times.

The least effective way to MASTER this material is merely to read the question and, without any effort, immediately turn the page to the answer.

You can't COGNITIZE the material in just one time through the check up questions. You only LEARN the material after several runs. The story teaches IN to your brain. The check up questions take OUT what you learned. They are *engineered* to help you make the proper adjustments.

It really is OK for you to get the answers to the check-up questions wrong on the first time through. That is typical.

Read the book again, after you go through the check-up questions a few times. Then wait a few days and read it again. The more you study the material, the faster you will grow.

Remember, I have not completed teaching until you are able to answer all the check up questions correctly. Thanks for helping me do a good job!

JIM

CHAPTER 1

THE FUNDAMENTALS

CBR

In days of old everyone believed the earth was flat. They behaved accordingly. How could they do otherwise?

People have CONCLUSIONS
that gives rise to BEHAVIORS
which yield life's RESULTS!

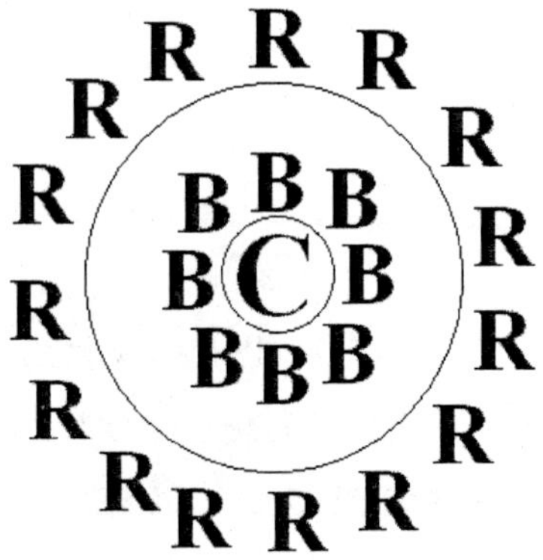

Conclusions are *absolutely and inseparably* linked to behaviors.

Behaviors are *absolutely and inseparably* linked to results.

Therefore, *conclusions and results are inseparably linked.*

If you wish to improve the results in your life, why not go directly to upgrading your conclusions?

When we try to modify another person's behavior, we become the disciplinarian.

If we help to change the other person's belief, he or she becomes self disciplining!

You cannot give away that which you do not have. Work on your own "Mental Fitness" first!

KNOWDOBE

People first learn COGNITIVELY. They come to know something new that they did not know before the learning experience. Learning NEW information is the beginning of real and permanent change.

Secondly, they learn AFFECTIVELY. They stop making the behaviors based on the old belief and implement the behaviors associate with the new conclusion, or belief… It takes time.

Thirdly, they learn EFFECTIVELY. They increase their command of the new belief by helping other people learn these new beliefs.
TO KNOW   TO DO   TO BE – "**KNOWDOBE**"

This book is *engineered* to help you learn to KNOW a dynamic *new belief* that improves your life.

PHILOSOPHY OF LIFE

There is a distinct system we use to develop and continuously update our philosophy of life. It begins with an **EVENT**, a feeling, something you imagine, a behavior you observe, taste, hear, feel, smell or get an idea about. Simply stated, an event is something that happens. Our mind records everything that happens in what I call a 3D mode - forming a visual, auditory, and emotional interactive record permanently retained for all time. It is recorded in your brain. It becomes a file or part of a program in your "LIFE OPERATING PROGRAM."

THE INTERESTING THING IS,.. WE CAN *DECIDE* TO INPUT CORRECT INFORMATION AND THEN *DECIDE* TO USE THAT NEW AND CORRECT INFORMATION INSTEAD OF THE OLD.

EVENT

Analysis

THOUGHT

Comparison

CONCLUSION

Selection

ATTITUDE

Prioritizing

VALUE

Compiling

PHILOSOPHY OF LIFE

For the sake of discussion, an event is something we agree has a start point, an end point, and whatever OCCURS, in between those two points, we establish as the information to evaluate. Whether we realize it or not, we think about the event. We unconsciously and systematically make an ANALYSIS of what happened. Through inductive and deductive reasoning, we work at it until we reduce what happened to a complete **THOUGHT**.

Each of our thoughts about events that have occurred throughout our entire life is separate from the others – like a single computer file!

As our mind manages all this information, we subconsciously begin to compare all our thoughts to determine which thoughts relate to other thoughts. The mental process of assimilating related thoughts permits us to formulate a **CONCLUSION** – like a computer folder!

Just as, in the formulation of a conclusion, we sifted through many thoughts, our mind makes a decision that some of these conclusion folders make up a unique larger folder of information that is related and compatible. We subconsciously SELECT from many of these similar or related conclusion folders to form an **ATTITUDE**. Attitudes enable us to form a more solid general position from which to react or respond to similar situations in our life.

Again, an ATTITUDE is a **previously developed position** enabling a person to react or respond somewhat automatically to recurring life situations - without having to stop and think through everything each and every time a similar circumstance or situation occurs. We gradually program ourselves to operate with less effort and energy.

To understand the word **VALUE,** we merely think of PRIORITIZING, or ranking our attitudes - with the attitude having the most meaning, importance, significance, or merit, at the top of the list and the attitude of least importance, worth, or utility, at the bottom.

Normally people think attitudes are our values! **I believe that perception is incorrect**. I believe our value system operates somewhat independently from our attitudes. When most people talk about their values, they are really talking about their conclusions or their attitudes. Our attitudes change very little as the value, **or the order of ranking** on the priority list, changes constantly. We change the ranking order of our attitudes with each new situation presented.

Today we are impeccably honest - but tomorrow, in a different situation, with different circumstances, we think it is better to withhold the truth or even tell a little white lie. Our conclusions and attitudes did not change - just the situation.

Our **PHILOSOPHY OF LIFE** is the final result of analyzing events and happenings to form thoughts, comparing thoughts to decide our conclusions, selecting conclusions to form attitudes, ranking an attitude to establish value, and COMPILING all of our attitudes into a master life plan. Our philosophy of life is the integrity ***program*** that generates our character and reputation. If we are to change character, we have to start examining the information that made up the events and thoughts in our early life.

The dictionary definition of PHILOSOPHY is:

1) The study and knowledge of the principles that cause, control, or explain facts or events.

2) Study of the basic principles of a particular field of knowledge.

3) Practical wisdom that comes from knowledge of general laws and principles.

4) A system of general beliefs or views.

5) Serenity, composure.

SPECIAL WORDS

BELIEF; The mental acceptance of the truth or actuality of something we give credence to, have faith in, conviction about, or are persuaded to accept as opinion. The act of the mind, or the mental ascent to something as being true. Beliefs are based on reasoning or fruit of authority - and not uncommonly *the fruit of prejudice, myths, or invalid sources* of information that are incorrect or filled with error data.

FAITH is acting on a belief trusting the belief to be true and trustworthy.

TRUST is an assured reliance, often instinctive, upon the truthfulness, honesty, or uprightness of another person or a belief.

CONVICTION is a *confirmed belief or conclusion* arrived at through reasoning - confirmed by real proof from unquestionable evidence. Conviction is grounded in reality and factual information that can be relied upon regardless of circumstances or the situation. Convictions are embraced only after the result of careful examination of new information.

Convictions are reliable - while beliefs, which we inherited from culture, are unreliable program files to use in our Life Operating Program – LOP.

I like to gain a conviction that I have labored over until I am confident I have it right. Convictions stand the test of time.

After mastering the material in this book, I hope you, too, will question everything you came to believe since you were a child!

PARADIGMS

A Paradigm (PAIR-A-DIME) is a SHARED or MODEL perception.

If I asked: "What is the most famous fast food restaurant in the world?" most people would say "McDonalds." Ninety of 100 people would give that same answer. They would share in that conclusion. Those 90 people make up what is called a paradigm. The other 10 per cent make a second paradigm.

If I asked, "What significant event happens when a person reaches age 16?" 50 per cent would say: "getting a driver's license." Thirty per cent would say: "Dating." And 20 per cent would list one of several other conclusions. There is more than one paradigm about what is the most significant thing that happens at age 16.

Because more people share the same conclusion or perception about the "driver's license" than those with the "dating" as their perception, the drivers license paradigm is stronger than the paradigm about dating.

Before people start to learn the subject of "Mental Fitness," many unknowingly (I repeat unknowingly) think, believe, or have the conclusion "other people or outside situations make them mad and angry or sad and depressed." I intend to prove they may unknowingly have this conclusion – even though they may at first deny it.

That is their first perception; this is what they think before they learn new information.

After they complete this learning experience, they no longer believe (unknowingly) that others or outside situations control their emotions.

Their first perception contained some error information. We call it the "**BEFORE**" or "OLD" conclusion. Their second perception contains reality information. We call it the "**AFTER**" or "NEW" conclusion.

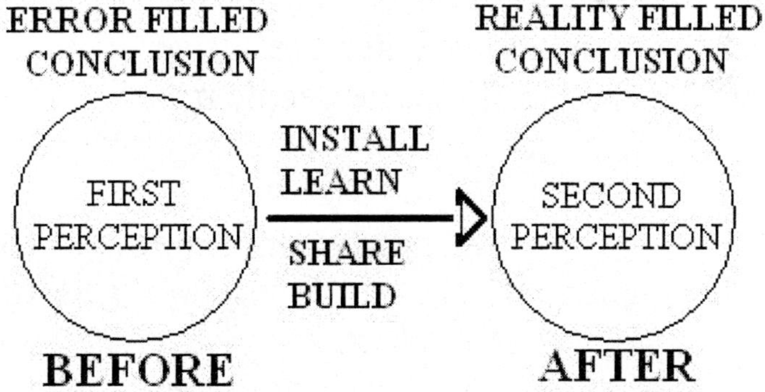

The purpose of this book is to share new precepts and concepts that will enable you to communicate more effectively with yourself and then with others.

When parents become more "Mentally Fit," they naturally discipline their children more appropriately!

NOTES OR QUESTIONS

CHAPTER 2

THE STORY

When I lived in Gresham, Oregon, I had a neighbor a couple doors away whose mother came to visit. They both came over to my house. And, when the mother started to express her feelings, she said:

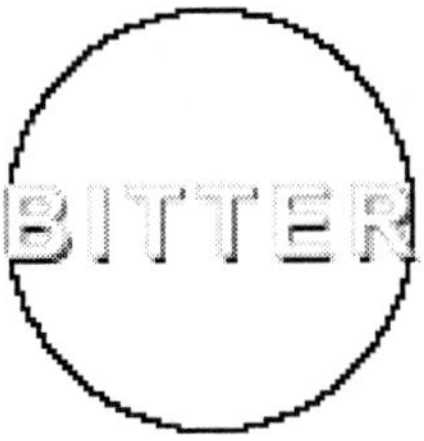

"Well I don't care what anyone says,... I'm bitter... I'm 53 years old... I've been divorced three times and I don't have any plans of getting married again. Marriage is just too much of a hassle.

The first time I was married for 10 years and he left me with two children to raise by myself. There wasn't enough child support money, so I had to work

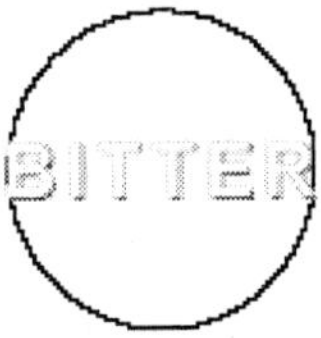

(1) in a restaurant to make a living. I certainly wasn't (2) prepared to go out and get a good job. I'd been raising children - not going to college like he was. I was really caught flat footed.

The second guy, I was only married to for two years and he took off too.

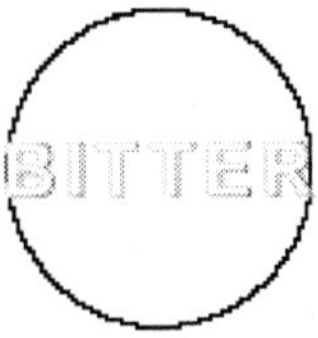

The third guy only lasted (1) three months... and I threw him out before that (2) situation went sour - like the other two. (3)

I think life is tough. It's really a dog eat dog world. Only the strong survive. If you don't climb over people to get to the top, you don't get there. And that baloney about how you can learn to live a happy life and have a happy family is a bunch of bunk.

I'm a bitter person. The only retirement I have is social security and it's too late to start over. I don't expect anything from anyone any more.

You can't even trust people any more. If you leave your car unlocked, they rip you off and take you for everything you have. This world is a nasty place. I don't care what anyone says, I'm fed up with life and the whole mess."

I said, "Perhaps if we talk a bit I can help you overcome some of your bitterness."

She said, "I'll tell you what would help me overcome the bitterness. You take those three guys out and horse whip them for what they did to me. They are the ones who made me bitter. You take care of them and I will really be a happy person."

I said, "Well if we talk awhile, and I can teach you something about mental fitness, maybe you won't think like that any more, and you can feel better about life."

We talked for quite a while. I was able to obtain some more information about her life that I want to share with you.

I want you to see how her behavior was working exactly the opposite of her intent. It was the way she thought, or her thinking, that was her problem - not her three husbands or other people.

In order to explain these phenomena, I'm going to dramatize her story a little bit to emphasize the dynamics of the problem. The stories will make it easier for you to remember.

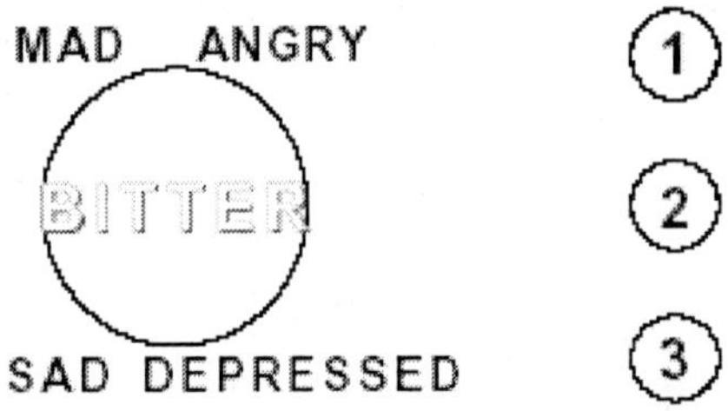

I drew a circle. In the circle I wrote the word BITTER. This was the word she used to describe her feelings and the way she perceived life. It wasn't my word.

Then I wrote the words MAD, and ANGRY, above the circle. Below it I wrote SAD and DEPRESSED. I did so to point out what she was **DOING** in the bitterness.

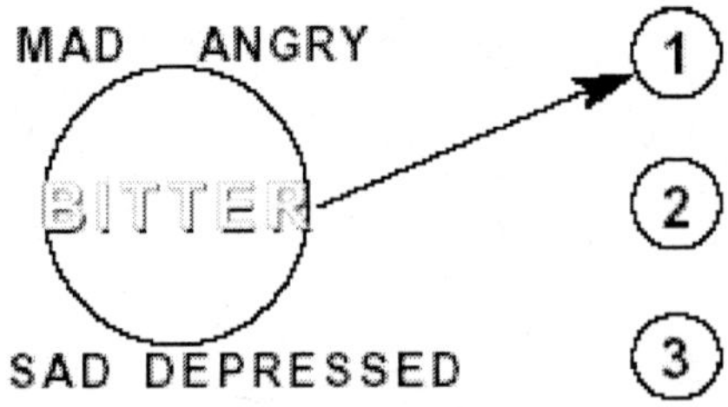

In other words, I divided the circle into some of the **COMPONENTS** of the bitterness.

This way we can better understand the functions of bitterness - or what she is doing in the process of her interactions with other people - her behaviors.

Then I drew an arrow, from the circle with BITTER in it, out to husband number 1.

When she met her first husband, she knew INSTANTLY that he was the one. He was tall and handsome. He wore a three piece suit with a white

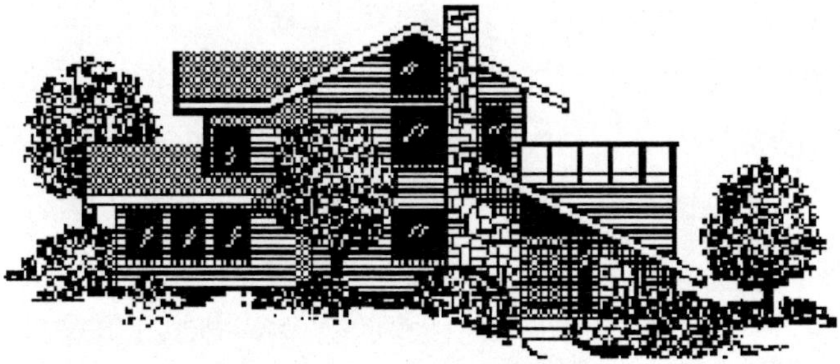

shirt and tie. He was a college graduate with the promise of becoming a big executive. She had visions of living in a big beautiful home with two cars in the garage, a nice

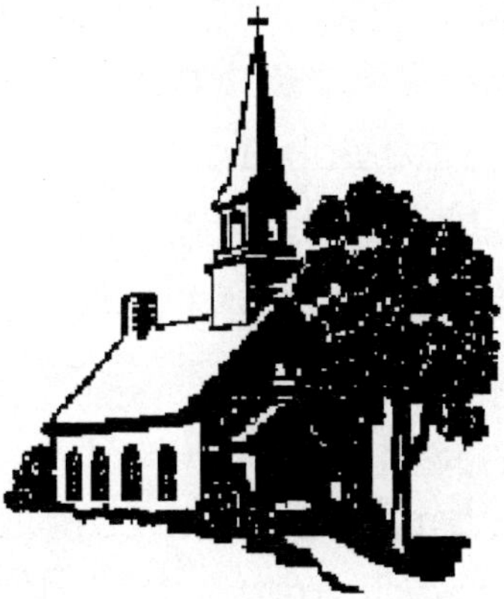

swimming pool in the back yard, and frequent trips to Hawaii, the Caribbean, and Europe. They would be an upper middle income family who went to church each Sunday with their little daughter and a son - who would be a chip off daddy's old block.

They had a story-book romance, a story-book engagement, and a story-book wedding in the story-book little church down the lane.

Then, after a few months, they bought their house on story-book lane. In a few years, they had a story-book little girl and a story-book boy. They became a story-book family.

Every story-book morning, after the family shared a story-book breakfast, father got in the story-book car and headed off down story-book lane to the story-book office. There, with all his story-book wisdom, he solved story-book problems for the story-book people all story-book day.

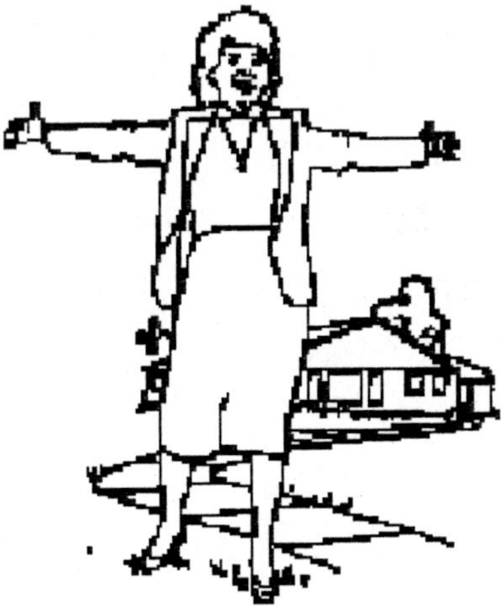

Every story-book evening at exactly six o'clock, father came driving back down story-book lane to his story-book house. The sun was setting beautifully in the trees behind the house. His wife was waiting, with her arms outstretched, to welcome him home with a story-book kiss. He was home,.. where the cares of the world would be left behind,.. and the family would be "together" again.

The children always waited to run and jump into father's arms. It was the highlight of their day.

The dog would get so excited he would bark,.. squeal with delight... and jump all around. The dog was glad to see his master too.

Then the family would go into the story-book house and sit down at the story-book table to eat their story-book meal. It was easy for mother to fix a nice five course meal as the children always helped her around the house.

The children always kept their rooms clean, never got dirty, got all A's in school, never said a bad word, and went happily to their story-book bed each night - without having to be told.
While they ate dinner, each family member, in proper turn, would tell the others what their day was like. The others said encouraging things like, "wonderful," "oh how great," and "isn't that marvelous."

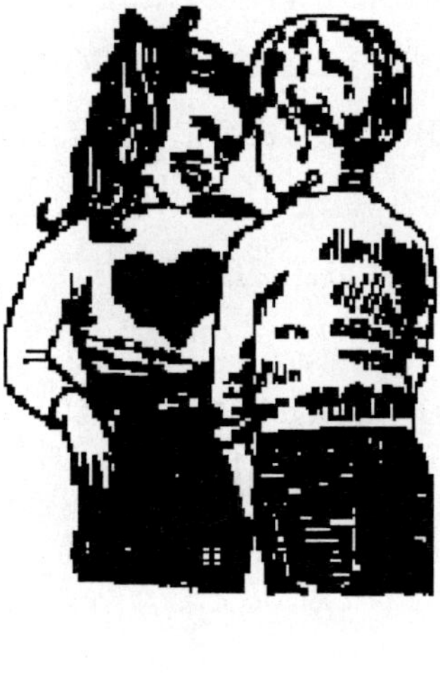

After the meal, the children would carry the dishes to the kitchen. Mother would wash, father would dry, and they would all sing camp songs in harmony.

Then father would take the children on his lap in front of the roaring fireplace, and read them a story, from a story-book, about another story-book family... while mother smiled and did some knitting.

After the children were in bed, father and mother would sit together on the couch and chat about things or discuss family matters. They wanted to assure they were in agreement on everything so the family would always run smooth - in a story-book way.

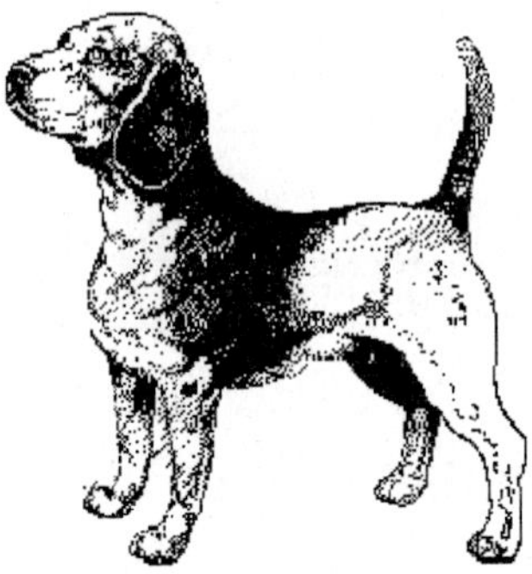

Then one evening, at six o'clock, mother was standing at the door with her arms outstretched and waiting to take father into her welcoming embrace. The kids were crouched waiting to leap into Father's arms. The dog was excited and wagging his tail.... but, at six o'clock, father didn't show up...?

By 6:15 mother’s arms were tired and the kids couldn't crouch poised to leap into father's arms any longer - as their legs were getting cramped up a bit. The dog had stopped barking and wagging his tail and looked quizzically at everyone, as he couldn't understand the situation.

By 6:30 our story-book tale started to fall apart. Mother was alarmed that something might have happened to father. She became concerned.

The children began to complain that they were hungry. They were saying things like, "Mom, the food's getting cold. Mom, the candles are burning down." "Mom, my stomach is growling. Mom, let's eat,.. Dad will be home in a little bit."

The dog started howling as he could not stand the discord.

By 6:45 mom and the kids gave up and started eating their cold food - but the mood was gloomy.

At seven o'clock when father drove up in the story-book car,.. mom was really mad at him. When he got in the house she said, "I'm really mad and it is your fault. You should have called and said you would be late. I was worried about you."

Components: getting mad, angry, sad and depressed indicate what she was DOING in her bitterness

He said, "Hon, your right. It's my fault you're mad at me. I apologize. I promise I'll never be late again."

So they were happy again - in a story-book way.

But, two weeks later, father was late again - and hadn't called this time either.

This time mother was sad. She had a tear in her eye. She said to father, when he came in the house: "I'm really sad and it's your fault. I worked hard to fix a really nice meal, and get everything ready just for you, and you don't even care about me enough to call on the phone to say you're going to be late. I'm really broken hearted, and it's entirely your fault."

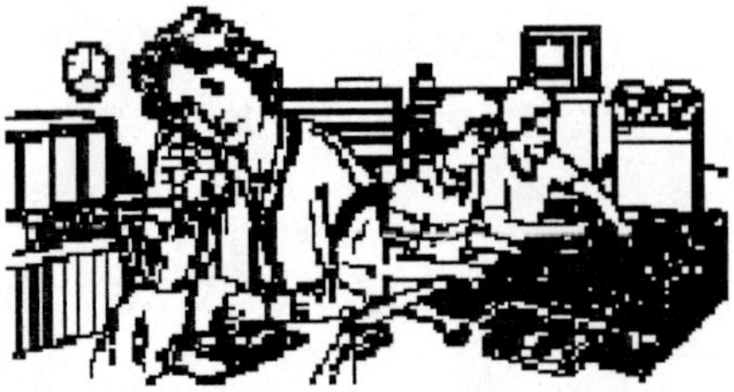

He said, "Hon, you're right. It’s my fault again. I accept all the blame for everything. I'm truly sorry I made you sad. I promise I will never be late again.

But, with every new promotion in the company, it seemed father had more and more responsibility and more obligations to the company. His meetings and appointments were not always finished right on time. He began to come home late more and more often. Many times he couldn't get out of the meetings even to make a phone call to tell her he would be late.

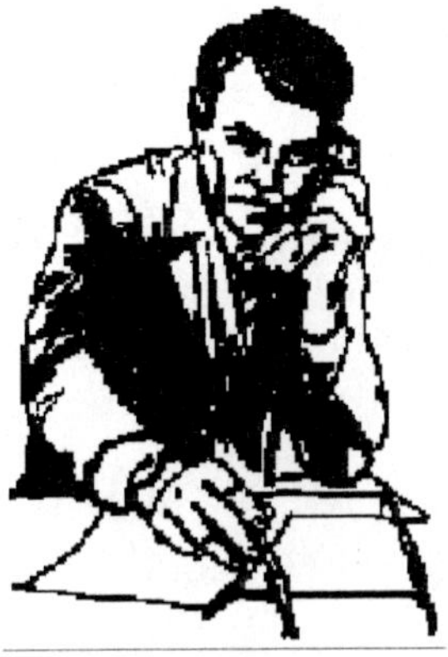

So, each time, when he got home, she was more mad and angry. She said he didn't love her any more. All he cared about was his company.

He argued that he did love her more than the company, but he couldn't promise, anymore, what time he was going to be home.... he told her that when he was late, they should go ahead and eat without him.

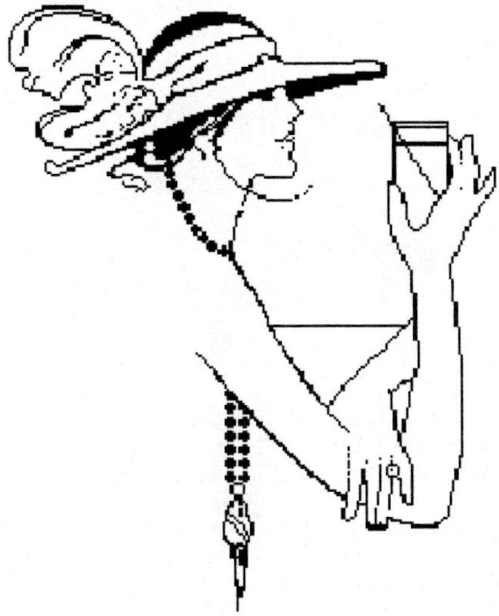

He began to travel, take clients to dinner, attend seminars, conferences, and conventions,... leaving his wife at home to tend to the children.

At night, when he was gone, she would lie in bed, in the silence, and feel lonesome and depressed. She had no adult to relate with. There was nothing to do and no one to talk to.

When he came home she would say, " Hon, I'm depressed, and it's your fault. You're not married to me any more. I believe you're married to the company. The company means more to you than me or the children.

He would argue that he had told her before that he did love her, but he absolutely had to work to put the roof over their heads, the food on the table and clothes on their backs. He wondered why she couldn't understand that she was putting undue pressure on him - and it made him mad. He was getting pressure at work and pressure at home, too.

Father's secretary could see clearly that he really loved his family... and that he also loved the people in his company.

It appeared to her, that every time his wife called him, she was either MAD, SAD, ANGRY, or DEPRESSED about something. His wife was constantly blaming him for all her bad feelings.

The secretary certainly loved her boss. One day, after seeing how bad he felt about his wife's phone call, she put her arm around him and said, "You know, I think you're a really great man."

Some things at the office began to look a little better than some things at home. Home just wasn't the same old story-book place any more.

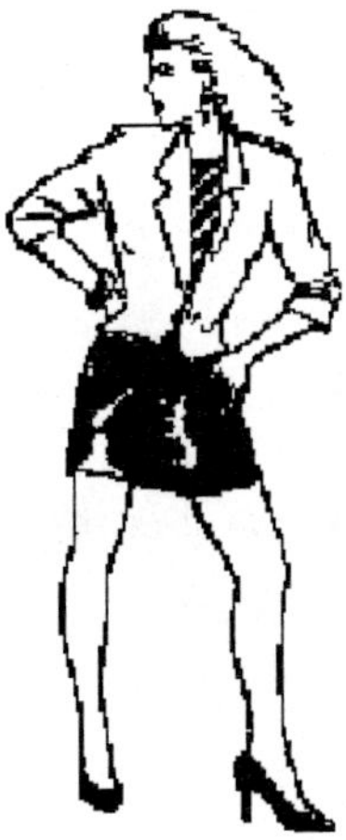

He loved his wife and wanted her to be happy. But it appeared he'd failed. He did not want the kids to grow up in an atmosphere of constant arguments and disharmony. He wanted his life to be happy, too.

The only solution he could see was divorce. He thought he had tried every way he knew to solve the problems, but nothing had worked.

So he told his wife, "Hon, I really love you and hope you can find someone who can make you happy...

“I'm leaving. I'll send you money every month to help you.

I just can't take the **PAIN** of our relationship any more."

After he packed his story-book suitcase, he left with his promise to send her some story-book money every story-book month.

Well, this really made the wife bitter. She had no job skills, was 32 years old, had two kids to support, and the story-book money, sent by that ©*#@ husband #1, just didn't make ends meet. Since she hadn't really developed any professional job skills, she was forced to take a job as a waitress. She really felt dumped on. She was certain the secretary had stolen her husband... She hated him for what he had done to her.

She had been divorced for three years, when she met her second husband. She knew INSTANTLY he was the one. She was sitting on a blanket, having a picnic with her children, near the woods, when a "Knight" came riding over the crest of this hill on a big white horse.

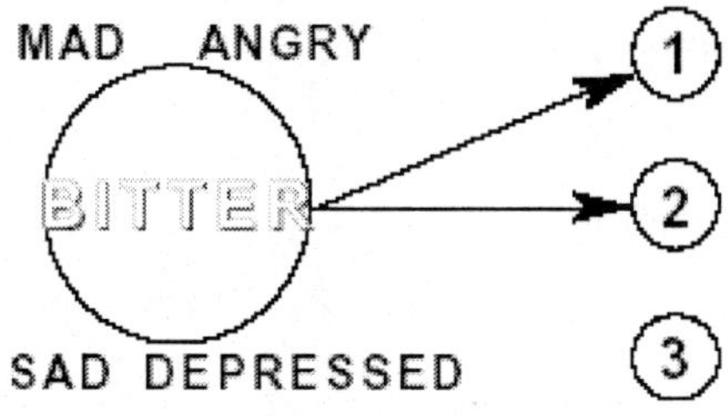

His dazzling chrome plated armor was shining in the sun. He carried a flag flying from the tip of the lance he was holding upright in his stirrup. The flag flying from the lance said: TRUTHFUL, HONEST, LOYAL, CHEERFUL, THRIFTY, BRAVE, CLEAN and REVERENT.

She knew that... here was a man who would never abandon her or treat her unkindly - as he was truly a man sent by God to rescue her from all the perils and bitterness of life.

And of course HE, being a knight, could not resist rescuing this beleaguered damsel from the terrible struggles of life. Besides, he thought she was super good looking - and of course the children needed a knightly father image to follow.

They were married privately in a small church.

Things went fine the first glorious year. Then one day, at six o'clock, he didn't show up on time for dinner. He came home late from training... that all knights have to do... and he had neglected to send her a message that he might be late. She met him at the door and told him, "I'm really mad and it's your fault. You should have sent a message you'd be late."

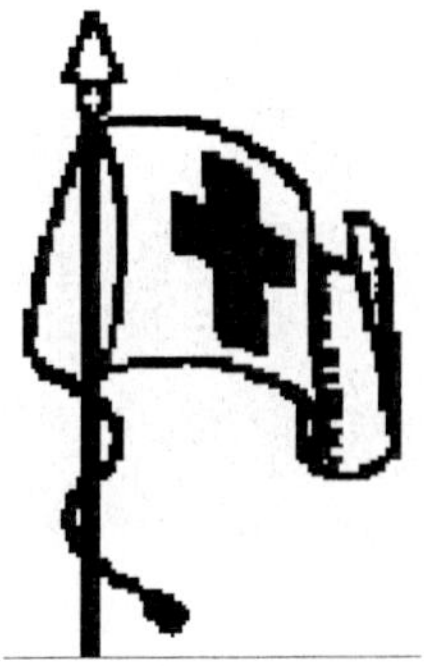

He said, " Hon, you're right... It's my fault you're mad and I apologize. I promise I'll never be late again."

And so, they were happy again in a glorious way. But, two weeks later, her knight in shining armor was late again - and hadn't sent word this time either.

This time mother was sad and had a tear in her eye. She said, "I'm really sad,.. and it's your fault. I worked hard to fix a really nice meal and get everything ready just for you.. and you don't even care about me enough to send a message that you're going to be late.... I'm broken hearted and it's your entire fault."

He said, "Hon, you're right. It's my fault again. I'm sorry I made you SAD. I apologize... I promise I'll never be late again."

But, as his career in knighthood escalated, he became more and more involved in doing his job. He came home at irregular hours. He had to spend more and more time in training to prepare himself for the crusades and the holy wars. He told her he couldn't promise her when

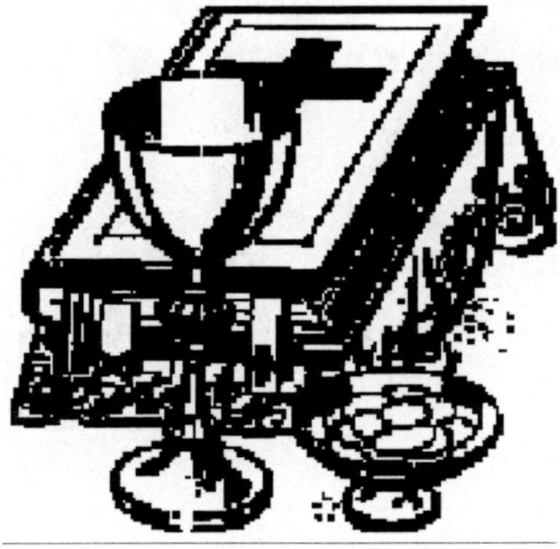

he'd get home. He would sometimes spend as much

as two weeks in the field on maneuvers... he told them to go ahead and eat if he wasn't there on time.

When he was away on maneuvers, she would lie in bed at night... all silent and lonely. She became depressed that she had no one to talk to. When he came home she said, "Hon, I'm depressed and it's your fault. You're not married to me, you're married to some QUEST. Your quest means more to you than me or the children."

Her knight would argue that he did love her, but he absolutely had to work to put the roof over their heads and the food on the table. He slowly began to develop some guilt feelings. Perhaps.. it really was his fault she was sad... He contemplated ways he could tell her that he really felt bad about how he had made her life even more miserable than it was before.

He felt such a strong calling to go on a crusade.... That kind of great sacrifice seemed to be a way of redeeming himself for all the pain he had inflicted upon her.

So he told her that he was divorcing her. He wanted her to find someone who could make her happy,.. and that she should go see husband number 1 about resuming payments of his story-book child support money...... as those weren't his kids to begin with. Oh... she was really BITTER now.

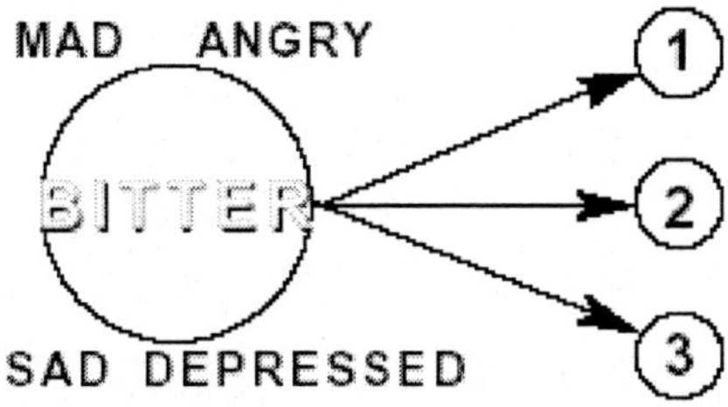

She was divorced from her second husband for two years when she met husband No. 3. And this time, she knew INSTANTLY he was finally THE one.

He came stomping down the street with those strong shoulders... bulging from the t-shirt with the sleeves torn off, his lunch bucket under his arm, his Levi jacket slung over his shoulder, hard hat cocked to one side and work boots on. She knew he was the one she should have married from the first. He was truly the "All American Standard Working Model." He believed in mom's apple pie, the American flag, and that hard physical labor was the most virtuous of all endeavors.

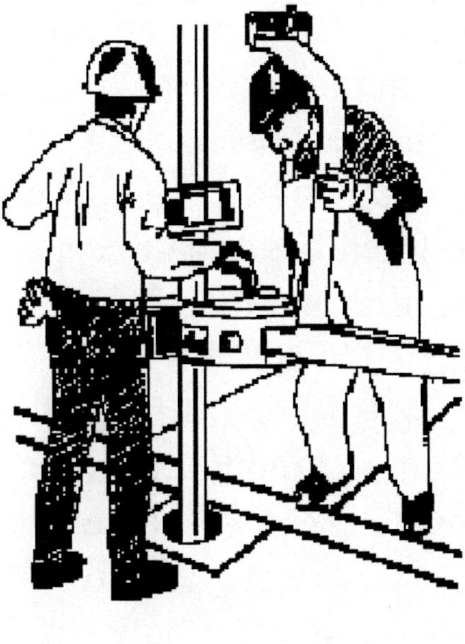

She realized that he might snore loudly, belly laugh at the beer commercials, guzzle beer and get mad all over the place if his meal wasn't hot on the table the moment he came home from work. But, he'd definitely be there - at home every single night watching TV.

They had been married 90 days when her tough loving "Hard Hat" said, "Hon, one of the guys on the crew is getting married. The boys and I are going to give him a real send off. I know your first two husbands never told you they were going to be late… So, I'm telling you now that I won't be home for dinner Friday night. In fact, I don't know what time I'll be home. If I remember right, the last time our gang did this, we ended up partying for the entire weekend! Oh, that was really a gasser. Let me tell you some of the stories from that one."

She said, "Whoa! Wait a second. I've been through this before... I can see with one eye what the story's going to be this time. The first guy married the company, the second married his QUEST,.. and you're going to start spending all your time with the BOYS..! Well, I'm not waiting around this time... Out of the house you louse... and don't come back!"

Well, now, that completes the story of how she came to be bitter. Let's analyze these situations and see if the analysis can help you to understand it is how she thinks.... and not the husbands... that are causing her problems.

First, I'm going to build an imaginary WALL, between her and the three husbands. I'm building the wall to isolate her from them, so she can "imagine" she will not ever again have any type of interactions with them. She is not going to speak to them, see them, hear from them, or in any way have contact ever again. The wall seals her off from them.

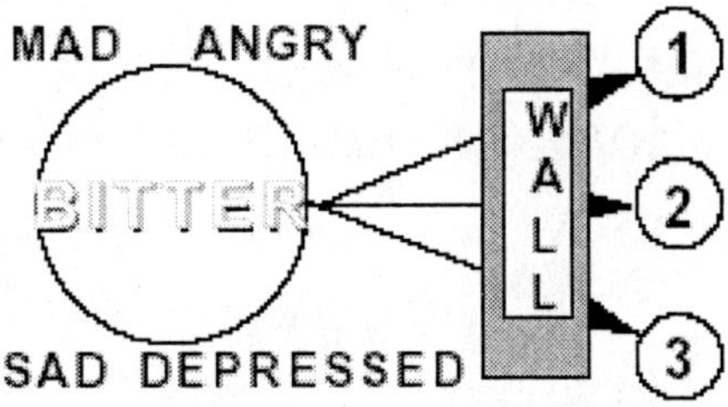

Once she is able to imagine being completely isolated, I ask her these 5 questions:

(1) Who is living in the bitterness?

(2) Who is experiencing the bitterness?

(3) Who is transmitting the bitterness?

(4) Whose life is being contaminated by the bitterness?

(5) Who loses?
Naturally the answer to all these questions is that.... **she is**..... Even she will admit to that.

Now the question: are the three husbands the real cause of her bitterness?

1. LIVING
2. EXPERIENCING
3. TRANSMITS
4. CONTAMINATED
5. LOSES

To answer that question, we will look at the 5 steps in what we call "PROCESS."

Everyone has NEEDS they want to get filled - or they encounter situations where they WANT to get their WAY about something. The words "Needs," "Want" and "Way" are really one and the same. They are the starting point for examining the process of how we interact. A person initiates some type energy or effort, to go after something, or uses energy or effort to influence a particular outcome to a situation.

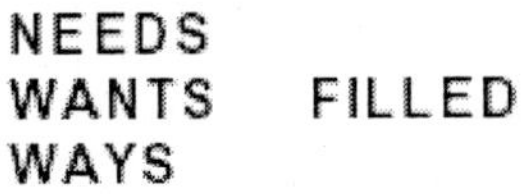

We develop a desire (NEEDS, WANTS, and WAYS) for something (STEP ONE), and then take some kind of **<u>action to FILL</u>** that desire (STEP TWO).

What she wanted, was for her first husband to come home at 6:00 every evening and have dinner with her and the children. There is <u>nothing wrong</u> with that desire. It is a legitimate thing for her to want. They both agreed, at the start of the relationship, that he would come home at 6:00. But when he didn't come home at 6:00, as he promised, what she <u>wanted... got blocked</u> off from being filled - BLOCKED BEING STEP THREE.

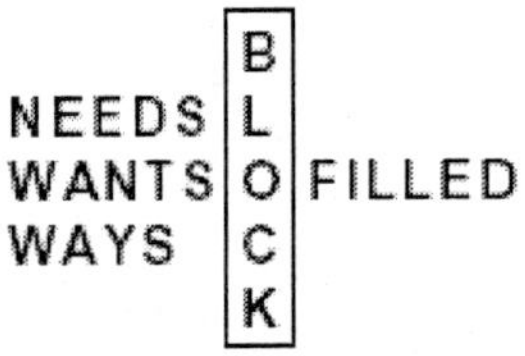

It is not a question of was she right or wrong, was it fair or unfair, was she justified or unjustified. The issue we are looking at is: "When she was blocked from getting what she wanted, what did she **do** - what PATTERN did she run?"

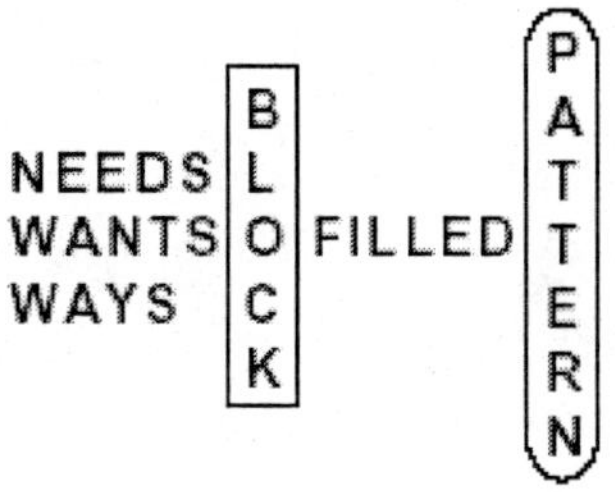

And the answer is... that she got bitter. That is to say, she got mad, sad, angry or depressed.

In this case we could say she took the "justified" route to being bitter.

She wanted him to come home in the evenings and spend his time with her and the children. There is **nothing wrong** with wanting that to happen. When he didn't come home (stayed at work, went traveling or to a seminar) she was blocked from getting what she wanted... and she blamed her husband for her bad feelings.

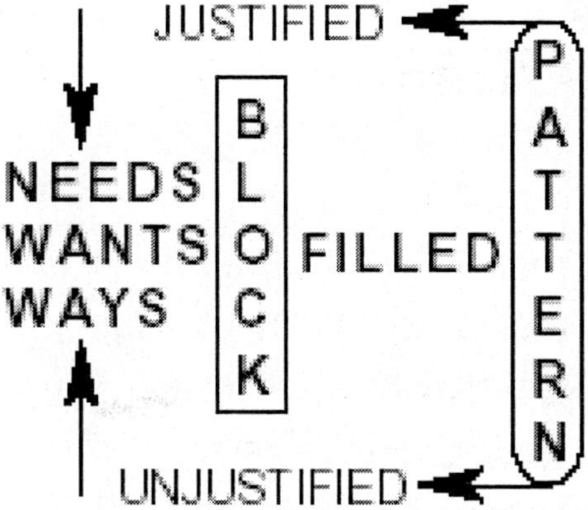

Again, we are not looking at this situation to see if it was fair or unfair, right or wrong, justified or unjustified. We are only looking at the process of what's happening in the interaction.

But people do not become angry only when it's fair... when they are right.... or when they are justified. They become angry when they don't get what they want.... If they don't get their way, they are angry. It has nothing to do with the situation - it has to do with how they think.

She began to build a pattern of becoming more and more bitter every time she was blocked from getting what she wanted. She started by getting mad. After some practice,.. she was able to get angry.

We are looking at the process of how people interact. The process has 5 parts that we are going to examine:

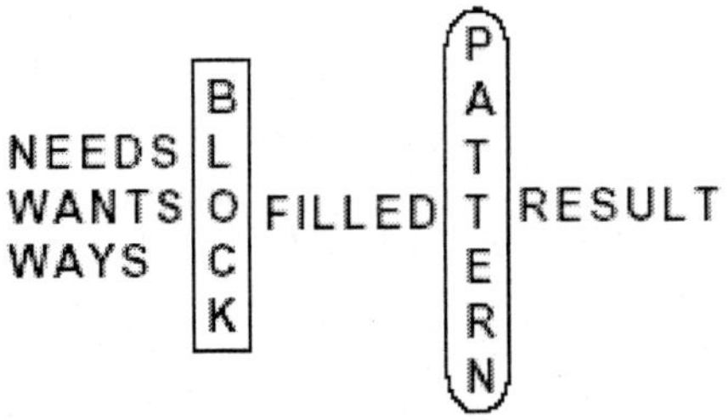

1. We generate our **NEEDS, WANTS,** or trying to have our **WAY** about something.
2. We determine a plan to get it **FULFILLED.**
3. We often get **BLOCKED** from having our wants filled.
4. We begin to run a **PATTERN** or build additional energy to try to knock down the block or in some way eliminate it. We run patterns whether we are justified or unjustified.

5. We get a **RESULT** - either pay a price or gain a reward for our efforts.

These 5 steps always follow the same sequence.

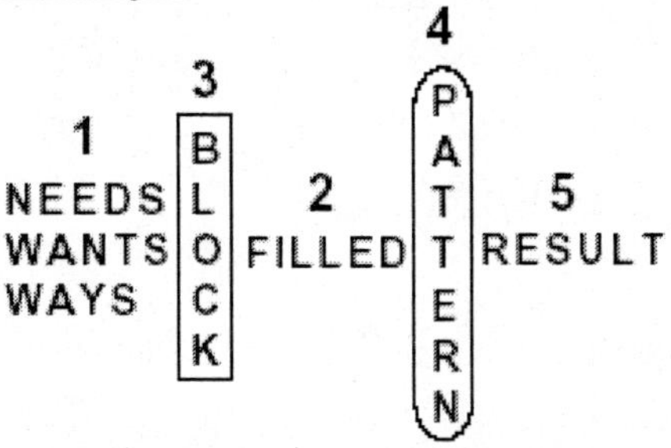

Some people tend to cling longer to their patterns if they think they are justified. Suppose I give this woman a large metal plaque to put on the wall. I say:

> "HEAR YE HEAR YE all nations, kindred, tongues, or people... Let it be known throughout the land, that this woman is completely justified in being bitter because of the terrible way these three men have treated her. In view of this, please do not disturb her, or encourage her to give up this bitterness, as she is completely justified in feeling bitter!

Even if she is totally justified, the 5 questions are still the same.

1. Who is living in the bitterness?

2. Who is experiencing the bitterness?

3. Whose life is being contaminated by it?

4. Who is transmitting it?

5. Who loses?

The answer is the same, SHE DOES!

In brief... it was her intent to have her husband come home on time... but, when he did not,.. she got mad at him. In reality, this behavioral display did not make him want to come home; it conditioned him to want stay away from her. It was an unknowing and unintentional self-defeating behavior.

It's as though I offered you a contract that said: "I'm willing to be your friend if you will be responsible for all my bad feelings. If you don't sign this contract, I'm going to be mad at you. It will be all your fault. In fact, any time I don't get my way, I'm going to be upset... and blame my upset condition on you."

Would you ever sign a contract like that?

You say you wouldn't because every time I wanted my way about something and you blocked me I would get mad, sad, angry or depressed and it would be your fault.... the only way you could stop me from becoming angry or depressed would be to let me have my way. You wouldn't think I had placed any value on you. You would exist only to please me.

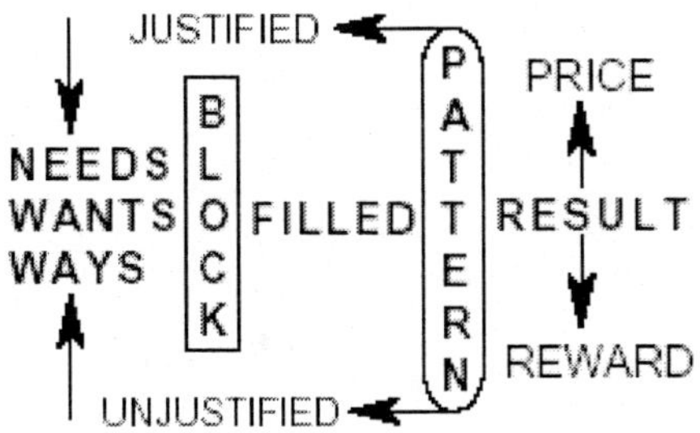

You say you wouldn't sign a contract like that... but, when is the last time you blamed your friend, spouse, your children, your boss, or someone else for your bad feelings? When is the last time your friend blamed you for their bad feelings? When is the last time one of the children got angry with you or their brother or sister and said their anger was the other's fault? It looks as if we might have the contract going already, don't realize it, and need to take a look at what we're doing to each other.

Each time the woman blamed her husbands for her bad feelings she was conditioning them to move further away from her... but she didn't realize what she was doing..... she was **not aware** that her behavior was functioning the opposite of her intent.

Let's look at some examples of what we are talking about, as we try to better understand the PROCESS of our interactions.

We will all go down to the local one-stop shopping center and set up our observation post near the candy section. We'll put some masking tape on the floor all around the candy section to assure we are all observing subjects in the same area. A little boy and his parents come into the area marked off for observation. The boy sees the candy. What is the first thing that happens when he sees the candy? He WANTS some... so he initiates some kind of action to get his want FILLED - such as pointing at the candy and saying:, "Mommy, Daddy, I want some of that candy."

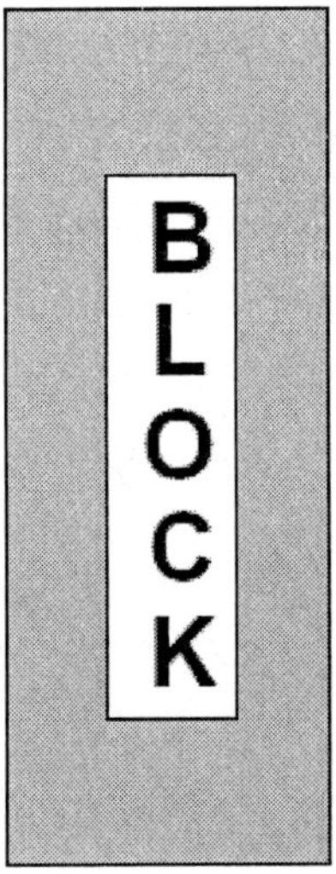

Mother and father now have a problem. No matter what they say - or how they say it - they are going to **BLOCK** the boy from getting his want filled.

They may say, "No! No, that isn't good for your teeth. No, you had some yesterday. No, we don't have time. No, we are in a hurry to get you a toy." They could say no for any reason and it wouldn't make any difference to the boy... and what he is doing.

If they say anything that BLOCKS the boy from getting what he wants, what is he going to do? He will run some sort of pattern - such as throwing a little temper tantrum or cry and sob his heart out.

What is father likely to do if the boy throws a temper tantrum? That's right, give the little boy a spanking right there on the spot. That is the RESULT (price) element we are talking about.

But, let's suppose they don't give him a good shot of discipline when he throws the tantrum. Suppose they are from a very *respectable* family and are aghast that their boy is acting like a little menace for their neighbors to see. They might run quickly to buy him the candy so he won't be so embarrassing to them. Is the boy now getting a reward for his behavior or is he paying the price?

It's easy to quickly say the RESULT he is getting today appears to be a reward. But, when he gets to be 20 to 40 years old, and married, and he doesn't get his way, what behaviors has he learned WORK to overcome the BLOCKS? And what price will he pay then, the loss of a spouse or a family living in pain? What are the parents doing? Not intending to do,... but actually doing..?

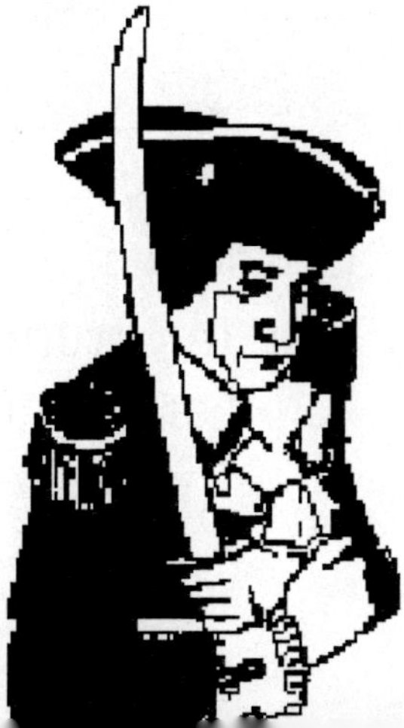

Here's another example. Father wants the house cleaned up by 9:00 a.m. each Saturday morning. He gives his orders to the family for the house to be ready for inspection. Mama and the children say: "Yes, sir!"

But... on Saturday morning,.. when father dons his military hat, puts his swagger stick under his arm and marches in to make his white gloved inspection,... mother is just rubbing the sleep from her eyes, and the children are still nestled snug in their beds,... with visions of sugar plums in their wee little heads.

Father wanted the house cleaned by 9:00 a.m. Now he's been blocked. The house hasn't been prepared for inspection. What pattern does the dictatorial father run? He punches mother out for insubordination and beats the kids until they are all hopping about quickly trying to get the house cleaned up for father.

What RESULT can father expect for running his pattern? Well - as soon as mother can - she's going to leave him. Sure, he may have been able to get the house cleaned up *for a while*, but what PRICE is he paying for a clean house if there is no harmony in the family?

When one of militaristic father's sons is on the playground and wants the swing that another child is in (and the other child doesn't get right out of the swing) the boy is likely to punch the other kid out. That's the pattern the militaristic father modeled for him - this is the way you act in order to get the things you WANT when you are BLOCKED.

Some people think that only other people can cause them to be blocked from having their wants filled and forcing them to run patterns. Let's look at this example:

You and I are following behind a car on our way to work. The driver in the car ahead of us has to cross the railroad track, get on the freeway and head down town to the office. He has only 15 minutes to get to work. It is critical he get to work on time - or he might be fired.

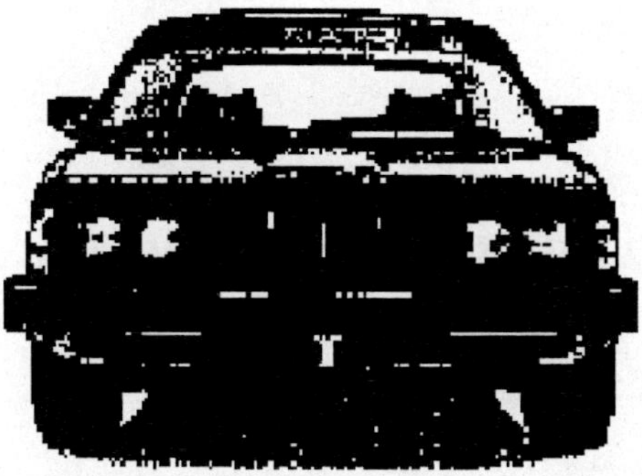

Just as the car approaches the railroad track, there is the *ding - ding - ding* as flashing lights on the crossbar come down - signaling the approach of a train.

Now, all we are doing is observing what the driver in the car is **DOING.** We do not consider if it is right or wrong, justified or unjustified. We are simply observing WHAT HE DOES.

As soon as the driver sees the crossbar block him from getting across the track, he realizes he may be late for work and in trouble.

As we observe, the driver goes slightly berserk in the car... he pulls his hair, pounds the steering wheel and finally crosses his fingers - in hopes that it is a fast AMTRACK passenger train. **But it's not**! Coming around the bend are five engines hooked together... pulling 349 boxcars!

Oh, boy, now he is really smashing his hands on the dash and beating his head on the steering wheel. He is yelling and cursing at the engineer - generally leaving small bits of flesh all over the inside of the car (on all of the sharp projections) as he thrashes around.

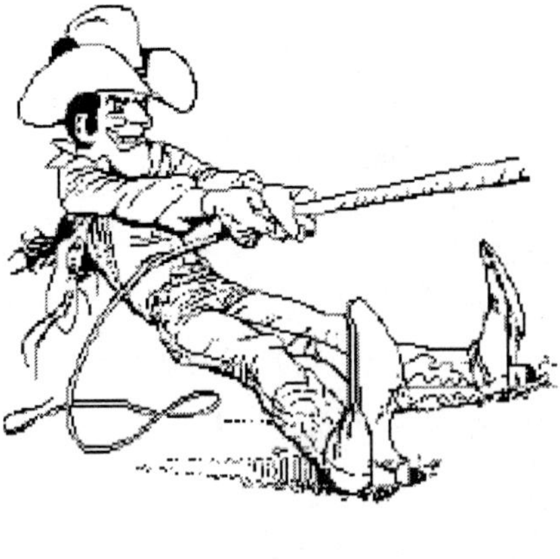

Finally, he sees the caboose coming around the bend. He starts the car, guns the engine and throws it in gear. But,.. the train slows. Now, he's waving his hands like a football fan yelling Go! Go! Go! Go! He's trying somehow to push the train past the intersection so he can get to work. The train stops.... with the caboose right at the center of the intersection. He holds his breath. He's stopped pounding his hands and waving. His eyes bulge and his heart pounds loudly.

Then, ever so... s. l. o.. w... l.... y,... the train starts to back up! Well,.. that's just too much for our hero. He jams the car in reverse and backs the car around, laying rubber all over the road with one wheel and slings gravel on the other motorists. He fish tails his way back up the road - heading toward the underpass that is back a mile or two.

What BLOCKED him was not a person… but <u>CIRCUMSTANCES</u>.

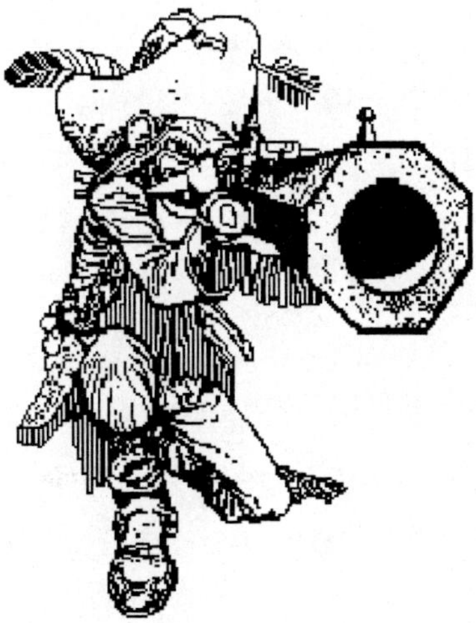

The issue is not whether he was justified. We are looking at what he is DOING or the pattern he is running - the feelings he is living in and shooting at others. Then we want to determine whether they are working for him in a productive way.... or against him in a non-productive way.

The woman, who was bitter, <u>did not intend</u> to make a series of behavioral displays that would condition her husbands to avoid her or move away from her. Regardless of her intentions, her behavior was doing just that. In fact, the more energy she put into getting them to come home, and stay home, the more her behavior worked against her.

Sometimes our behaviors do not reflect our intent. We need mental fitness education to see clearly how we are actually relating with others.

As I drew out the diagram, she said harshly to me: "You're making out like I'm the one that's crazy and not those three no good bums!"

I said: "No, I'm not trying to be a bad news person - telling you it was your fault at all. I am telling you that you are a person. As a person, there is nothing wrong with you. But you do have some bad conclusions that are causing you to unknowingly push away from you the things you are trying hardest to obtain. I want to help you to achieve understanding of the concept I'm trying to share with you, Let's use another illustration."

Let's say that we go to her and find out the qualities she would like to have in a husband - were she to marry again. Then we would go out and find at least nine men who fit that general description. We number them 4 through 12 - as shown in the graphics. Naturally, there are a lot of men that might meet the

4,5,6,7,8,9,10,11,12
RANDOM

qualifications, but these are men selected at <u>RANDOM</u> from among all those considered.

Now, we are going to take this person (who has a pattern of becoming BITTER whenever something blocks her from having her NEEDS, WANTS OR WAYS filled), and have her,... with this PATTERN, marry,.. let's say,.. number 9.

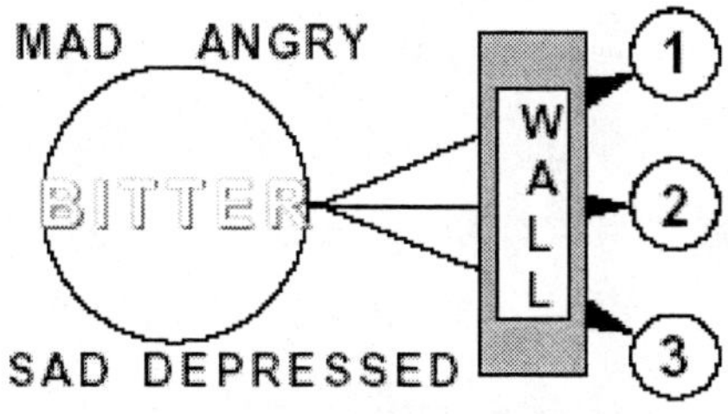

In this new relationship, the first time a situation occurs, where it is important to her to have HER way, and he says, No! - <u>what will this person with this pattern **do**</u>?

Regardless of whether she is justified or unjustified, this person, with this pattern, will become BITTER. And, when this person with this pattern gets BITTER, who will this person blame?.. Old number 9 of course!

It would be safe to say, that although she's never met No. 12,... were she to marry him, it would also be his fault that she is BITTER!

In reality, it's not the fault of any number, 1 through 12, that she is bitter. Her pattern is not the fault of others. It is something she is <u>doing</u> based on her beliefs – whether she is aware of her real beliefs or not.

Well, if it's not the fault of OTHERS, then whose fault is it?

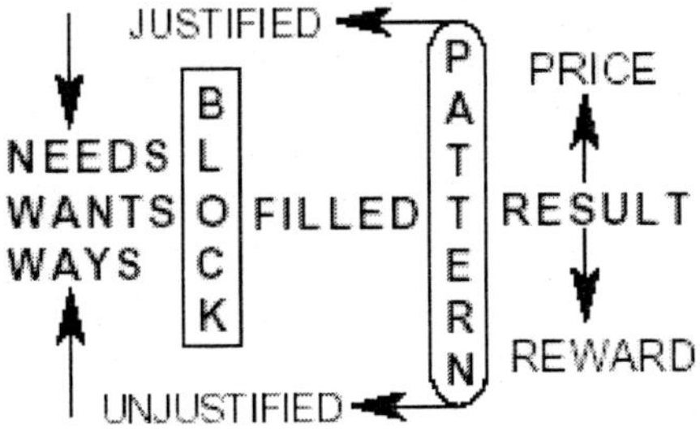

It's easy to draw a conclusion that it's her fault. But let's not think it's her fault. We can only say, it's still her responsibility. Let me explain: if it's her fault, what is she GUILTY of? It's certainly not her intent to do things that cause pain in her relationships. She is **not aware** that what she is DOING conditions others to avoid her! She is not aware that blaming others for her bad feelings, attempting to have her way, works the opposite of her intent.

In fact, the harder she tries (getting more angry or depressed) to make her husbands come home, the more they're likely to avoid her!

She has NOT LEARNED HOW to relate more effectively. If she just doesn't know, what is she guilty of? NOT KNOWING - she knows not what she is doing.

Can we really condemn someone who just simply... does... not... know...? Should we shun and avoid her, when what she really needs is for us to love her and teach her so that she can become aware.

If she learns to be more mentally fit, could she change her THINKERTOY so that she is able to choose to stop the self-defeating behavior and act in a way that does not push others away from her? To actually behave more according to her intent...!

What I'm saying is that any person who has any pattern will normally interact with everyone the same way - it is the way they unknowingly use a conclusion in their Life Operation System.

Conclusions must change for the behaviors to transmit loving intent in a way to gain the result the person already desires. **Love is not an intention - it is a behavior -** coming from a new and more mentally fit conclusion.

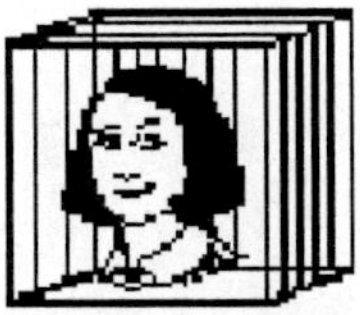

4,5,6,7,8,9,10,11,12
RANDOM

It's as if the woman lives in a cage of bitterness. In her mind, other people made her bitter. She thought she was trapped in the bitter feelings. She thinks other people MAKE her mad, angry, sad and depressed... and control her happiness.

As long as she thinks this way she's trapped ... in the cage of bitterness.

What is it that has to occur for her to escape the cage? She must cognitize what we are talking about.

She must become AWARE. She must understand. All these things are true, but in order to become aware, she must first... **<u>LEARN.</u>**

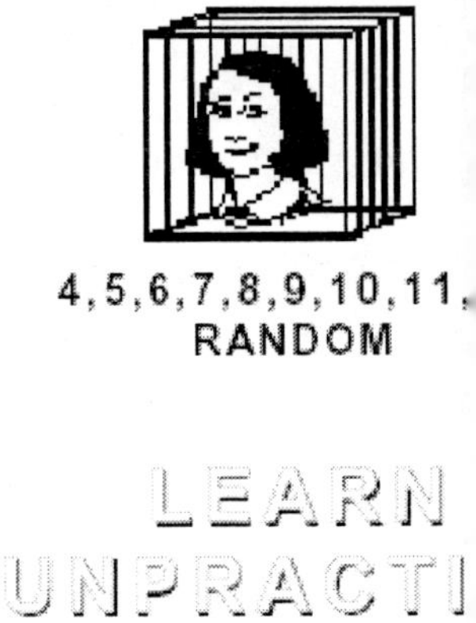

Being able to communicate effectively comes from an effective learning experience. You can't learn to become mentally fit by going out in the woods and banging your head against a tree. And you can't drink something from a bottle that enables you to think your way out of these problems. You must <u>learn</u>.... from a person who has learned. We have to pass it along!

The second thing a person must do, after they have learned, is to <u>unpractice</u>.

You are a person.... and NOT a pattern. You have the ability to step back and examine the process of how you interact with others. Once you learn the basic mental fitness concepts, you can easily determine if your behavior is producing the right results. You can change your conclusions so your behaviors more closely align with your intent. It becomes a natural process.

To AFFECT a change is a slow process. Just because you become aware of a conclusion that is driving your behavior, does not mean you are going to instantly stop running self-defeating patterns or instantly change to another behavior.

First, LEARN. Second UNPRACTICE. In another book we will provide you with information about CHANGING. It will help explain what you can do to accelerate your growth toward being a mentally fit person.

The last thing you need to do, to become a mentally fit person, is to go through an EFFECTIVE learning experience; help others to become aware, too.

THIS CONCLUDES THE PRESENTATION ON THE PROCESS OF COMMUNICATION.

IN THE NEXT CHAPTER YOU WILL GO THROUGH CHECK-UP QUESTIONS ENGINEERED TO EXPAND YOUR COGNITIVE UNDERSTANDING OF THE CONCEPT OF X TO N.

PLEASE READ THE INSTRUCTIONS ABOUT THE CHECK UP QUESTIONS, IN THE FRONT OF THE BOOK, BEFORE BEGINNING!

THANK YOU

Chapter Three

CHECK-UP QUESTIONS

QUESTION 1:

Why is it correct to say the results we get in our lives are linked directly to our conclusions or beliefs?

ANSWER 1:

Because the CBR graphic shown CONCLUSIONS are absolutely and inseparably linked to BEHAVIORS. It is impossible to have a behavior that does not come directly from a conclusion or belief.

Behaviors are absolutely and inseparably linked to RESULTS.

Therefore, RESULTS are absolutely and inseparably linked to our CONCLUSIONS. The words belief and conclusion can be used interchangeably.

In geometry we say if A = B and B = C, then A = C!

QUESTION 2:

What did Jim use the term "KNOWDOBE" to describe?

ANSWER 2:

The 3 methods of learning:

COGNITIVE - to learn to know something new.

AFFECTIVE - to change the behavior from the old conclusion to the new – to do

EFFECTIVE - to help others learn the new conclusion – to be.

QUESTION 3:

What is the most important thing Jim said about ATTITUDES in the section on Philosophy Of Life (POL)?

ANSWER 3:

An ATTITUDE is a ***previously developed position*** enabling a person to react or respond somewhat automatically to recurring life situations - without having to stop and think through everything each and every time a similar circumstance or situation occurs. Our Life Operating Program gradually programs ourselves to operate with less effort and energy.

QUESTION 4:

What is the difference between an ordinary conclusion and a CONVICTION?

ANSWER 4:

A CONVICTION is a *confirmed belief* arrived at through reasoning - confirmed by real proof from unquestionable evidence. Conviction is grounded in reality and factual information that can be relied upon regardless of circumstances or the situation. Convictions are embraced only after the result of careful examination of new information.

QUESTION 5:

What were the 2 questions Jim used to illustrate PARADIGMS?

ANSWER 5:

"What is the most famous restaurant in the world?"
"What happens when a young person turns 16?"

QUESTION 6:

What is the difference between “First Perception and Second Perception? – what were the ”special words” shown on the graphic?

ANSWER 6

BEFORE versus AFTER.

Error Filled Conclusion versus Reality Filled Conclusion.

QUESTION 7:

Was the word BITTER her word she used to describe her feelings, or was it Jim's word he used to label her as a bitter person?

ANSWER 7:

Her word she used to describe her own feelings.

She said: “I don’t care what anyone says, I’m bitter. I'm 53 years old... I've been divorced three times and I don't have any plans of getting married again. Marriage is just too much of a hassle.”

QUESTION 8:

The words mad, angry, sad, and depressed were called what?

ANSWER 8:

"**COMPONENTS**" of the bitterness

QUESTION 9:

Why did Jim take the components out of the bitterness?

ANSWER 9:

If you answered, "to show what she was feeling," you are partially correct – but Jim took the components out of the bitterness to show more what she was **DOING**.

She was getting mad, angry, sad, and depressed and then BLAMING others for the bad feelings she experienced – behaviors.

QUESTION 10:

In her "FIRST PERCEPTION" (before she became involved in a "Mental Fitness" learning experience), what kind of arrows were pointing from her to the three husbands? Were they blaming or pushing?

ANSWER 10:

BLAMING. In her first perception she thought other people caused her to be bitter. Yes, they were also pushing arrows – but she is not aware of that until she develops a second perception.

The conclusion she was using, in her Life Operating Program, was that her husbands were responsible for her feelings. So, therefore, she also thinks it was up to her husbands to make her happy, too.

QUESTION 11:

Was her conclusion that other people control her emotions a REALITY conclusion or an ERROR filled conclusion?

ANSWER 11:

An ILLUSION or ERROR FILLED conclusion. We say illusion because the information she is using to operate with is not true. It was induced into her Life Operating Program by culture. She only thinks it is true.

QUESTION 12:

In her SECOND PERCEPTION, were the arrows pointing from her to her three husbands blaming arrows or pushing arrows?

ANSWER 12:

PUSHING ARROWS. Constantly being mad, angry, sad and depressed and blaming other people for her bad feelings was unknowingly conditioning them to move away from her instead of closer. Her behavior was generating PAIN in the relationship.

I inform those I counsel about problems of divorce, they are not giving up each other, they are giving up the PAIN of the relationship.

When they married, they wanted to love each other and be happy together - but culture did them no favors. Culture programmed them to unknowingly generate pain. If they changed their programming, the pain would have gradually subsided, and love would have grown. But where do they go to get a programming change?

Long term counseling costs a lot of money! Most in the business focus on trying to teach people how to behave toward each other instead of going directly to the conclusions causing the problems. Counseling efforts are usually unsuccessful. Clients eventually get divorced.

QUESTION 13:

Was it her INTENT to condition her husbands not to want to come home?

ANSWER 13:

NO. In her mind she was trying as hard as she could to be happy. She could not understand why life was so painful.

Her behavior was unknowingly functioning the opposite of her intent.

QUESTION 14:

Since getting mad, angry, sad and depressed was working the opposite of her intent, why did she do it?

ANSWER 14:

She was NOT AWARE she was programmed defectively. She had not yet become aware, since she had not studied the subject of "Mental Fitness" in school (it is still not taught in schools), and had not learned it from her parents, religious leaders or her friends.

NOTE: She also was unable to learn it from her husbands as they were no better off than her. In fact, every time they took responsibility for all her bad feelings they were further disabling the relationship.

You cannot give away that which you do not possess.

QUESTION 15:

Who built THE WALL between her and the three husbands? Did she build it or JIM?

ANSWER 15:

JIM built the wall to ISOLATE her from her three husbands so he could ask her the five questions.

Who is LIVING in the bitterness?

Who is EXPERIENCING the bitterness?

Whose life is being CONTAMINATED by the bitterness?

Who is TRANSMITTING the bitterness

Who is LOSING?

QUESTION 16:

There are two routes from the block to bitterness – the JUSTIFIED route and the UNJUSTIFIED route.

Do people only run patterns when they are JUSTIFIED?

ANSWER 16:

NO. People run patterns any time they are blocked from having their needs, wants and ways filled.

QUESTION 17:

If we presented her with a plaque, medal or certificate, stating she was JUSTIFIED in being bitter (because of the way her three husbands treated her), would it alter her condition or improve her outlook on life?

ANSWER 17:

NO. In fact in might reinforce the problem.

QUESTION 18:

Do people tend to cling to bad patterns and feelings if they feel (or think) they are justified?

ANSWER 18:

YES. And they will continue to do so until they <u>learn</u> all their bad feelings are based on an ERROR FILLED conclusion. They have to face the facts presented in the five questions Jim asked when he built the wall to isolate her from her husbands, and decide:

These are my feelings.
I live in them by myself.
Blaming others does not change anything.
I'm the only one who can learn for me.
I am the only one who can change for me
I'm going to stop telling myself I have every right to be unhappy.
I'm going to quit expecting the outside world to make me happy.
Today is the first day of my liberated life.
I am going to learn to control my happiness.
I will not allow others (including motorists) to control my emotions.
I will always look around to make sure no one is looking before I run amok at railroad crossings.

QUESTION 19:

How many steps in PROCESS?

ANSWER 19:

FIVE.

QUESTION 20:

Do they always occur in the same SEQUENCE?

ANSWER 20:

YES.

QUESTION 21:

What is the FIRST step in process?

ANSWE 21:

Developing a NEED, choosing to WANT something, or trying to get your WAY in a situation. – what a person is after or trying to achieve.

QUESTION 22:

What STORY did Jim tell about the block to emphasize that sometimes a rational or logical answer does not stop people from attempting to get what they want?

ANSWER 22:

The BOY in the candy store.

QUESTION 23:

What story did Jim tell about the PRICE people could pay if they try to blast their way through the block to get their way.

ANSWER 23:

The story about the FATHER who wanted the house cleaned.

QUESTION 24:

What STORY did Jim tell to illustrate that not only people can block you off, but circumstance can also cause us to run patterns and experience distress?

ANSWER 24:

The man in the car at the RAILROAD CROSSING.

QUESTION 25:

When do people begin to experience distress?

ANSWER 25:

When anything or anybody BLOCKS them from having their needs, wants and ways filled.

I try to encourage people to distinguish between STRESS (a healthy force you use to exercise muscles) and DISTRESS – a negative emotional force generated by incorrect conclusions or beliefs!

I also encourage people NOT to say, “You are enabling that person.” Say, “You are DISABLING that person.” It makes a person more aware of what is going on.

QUESTION 26:

What were the numbers 4,5,6,7,8,9,10,11 AND 12 used to illustrate?

ANSWER 26:

To indicate PROSPECTIVE HUSBANDS selected at random, that people relate basically the same with everyone. Divorce and remarriage did not solve the problem. To show that it was not the fault of others that she was bitter.

QUESTION 27:

If it is not the fault of others, then whose fault is it?

ANSWER 27:

It would seem logical to say it is her fault.

But, in my opinion, no one is at fault. She was not aware her behavior was self-defeating.

But she alone is still responsible for her condition.

QUESTION 28:

If it was her fault, of what would she be guilty?

ANSWER 28:

To say it is her fault is to imply she is guilty of something.

The only thing she could be guilty of is NOT KNOWING!

QUESTION 29:

Not knowing what?

Answer 29:

Not knowing she has what Jim calls the eXternal conclusion that drives behaviors resulting from the input she received from culture to use in her "Life Operating Program."

We have the behavior to prove her conclusion that she thinks the eXternal world controls her emotions and determines her happiness. Up until now, she has not been aware she has been using that conclusion all her life. She may deny she has that conclusion. Again, the behaviors prove that is her conclusion. It is called unawareness.

When awareness finally comes to her, she may begin to think she needs to examine every conclusion she has inherited from culture to identify other beliefs that are faulty.

After reading this book you may find you get what I call a "BREAKTHROUGH." This usually occurs when you observe another person demonstrating they unknowingly have the X conclusion in operation.

QUESTION 30:

In her FIRST PERCEPTION, who does she think built the cage of bitterness or caused her to live in all the bitter feelings?

ANSWER 30:

Other people – and especially the three husbands.

QUESTION 31:

In reality, who built the cage?

ANSWER 31:

Thanks to culture, the X conclusion was responsible – not her.

QUESTION 32:

What is the first thing that must occur for her to get out of the cage?

ANSWER 32:

It takes a LEARNING EXPERIENCE that equips her with **NEW** INFORMATION that helps her recognize one of her Life Operating Program folders is filled with wrong information.

Nothing wrong with the computer – just a program that needs the virus removed. No matter how old she is, it's time to upgrade the system with "Mentally Fit" conclusions. The upgrade is available.

I hope this book helps you to build yourself an EDIT conclusion – one that goes through all your life operating program folders and identifies error data that may be affecting your life.

QUESTION 33:

After she LEARNS, understands and acknowledges she has the X conclusion, what is the second thing she must do to begin experiencing more joy and happiness?

ANSWER 33:

What I call UNPRACTICE, catch herself running the old blaming patterns. STOP… pause for a moment… remind yourself you have upgraded to the N conclusion (I am now INTERNALLY controlled and no longer believe I am EXTERNALLY controlled),… and START responding appropriately instead of reacting emotionally.

The good thing is, once people knew the world was round, instead of flat, they could never go back to believing it was flat again – and their behavior changed accordingly.

QUESTION 34:

If one group of people is experiencing condemnation toward any other group of people for any reason, who lives in the feelings of condemnation?

ANSWER 34:

THEY DO!

QUESTION 35:

Does this book only pertain to the problems of women?

ANSWER 35:

NO. It applies to every single person born into this world - regardless of whether they are male or female.

It is about the fact that everyone enters the world in the X mode and has to be "born again" into the N mode – "Know you not the Kingdom of God is within you?" "As a man thinks in his heart, so is he." "Forgive them for they know not what they do," are quotations that contain the elements of mental fitness.

Changing to the iNternal control conclusion allows people to be joyful, happy and successful in spite of the crazy world around them.

QUESTION 36:

Can anyone in the entire world LEARN *for* you or CHANGE *for* you?

ANSWER 36:

NO!

And, you cannot learn anything from someone who does not know about the X and N conclusions or about Mental Fitness!

You cannot teach that which you do not know!

If the blind lead the blind they both fall into the hole!

QUESTION 37:

If you do not liberate yourself from the X conclusion, what could you lose?

Answer 37:

Your friends, your job, your family and your happiness.

QUESTION 38:

How much time should I put into this effort?

ANSWER 38:

If you want to change your life for the better, invest the time required to master the content of this book. I suggest you read the book again and then go through the check up questions over and over until you answer every question precisely.

The more you understand the concept in the book, the quicker you should experience a BREAKTHROUGH.

That does not mean you are finished. It means you have arrived at the beginning. You have started to reverse negative growth and are on the way to being more effective.

There are so many things to learn about the "N" conclusion and EDIT conclusions. I get excited and want to share all that I have learned – but experience has taught me to take things one step at a time.

Will share more with you in the next book.

Please pass this book along to a friend.

Thanks!

JIM

ABOUT THE AUTHOR

J. W. "JIM" Campbell is originally from Shreve - a very small town near Wooster in the Northeastern Ohio.

A graduate of North High School in Columbus, Ohio, and The University of Nebraska at Omaha. Adjunct Professor at Seattle Pacific University for 6 years and teaching the subject of "Mental Fitness. He currently works as an author.

Jim is a retired U. S. Army infantry officer who served during the Korean War in one of the original Army Special Operation Units. He also served two tours in Vietnam with J3 on Joint Staff and as a District Senior Advisor in Bac Lieu Province.

Jim was selected to develop and implement the drug and alcohol abuse program for V Corps in Europe during the early 1970s. His resident rehabilitation program was selected by the United States Senate Drug and Alcohol Abuse committee as one of the 10 best programs in the world. This assignment got him started at developing the subject of "Mental Fitness."

After developing that program, Jim continued researching and developing the program while interacting with thousands of executives attending seminars provided by his company, Skills Of Communication (SOCNAT) in Portland, Oregon. As a community service project, he pioneered the development of a very long term "Mental Fitness" rehabilitation program at Oregon State Penitentiary.

The results of the program developed at Oregon State Penitentiary, after 20 years of collecting the research data, proved beyond any doubt recidivism was reduced to less than 15 per cent for those inmates involved in the program for at least one year. The technology of this new program focused on upgrading their basic beliefs.

The program cost is minimal because inmates facilitate the program under the supervision of existing trained correctional staff. The only cost is that required to start the program (one full week) and to continue with quarterly evaluations by highly trained SOC staff. This guarantees the quality of the program and allows correctional agencies to predict results.

Jim is also the author of the book "A Brief History of Early Westmoreland County, Pennsylvania." The book covers the period 1750 to 1775. It comes with a CD containing 10,000 names of the descendants of some of the earliest settlers to the south of Fort Ligonier.

Jim is presently writing books to provide people with more of his concepts about Mental Fitness: "EQUAL VALUE," "MAKING CONTACT SKILLS" and a book containing stories of "CHARACTER AND INTEGRITY" obtained from influential people Jim has met during his lifetime.

Jim and Jan are parents to 10 children, grandparents to 26.

He now writes as they travel in a motor home, currently located at Fort Huachuca, Arizona. Weather is great. Living among the soldiers is an honor. The SOS at the "Thunderbird" dining facility is scrumptiously nostalgic – thanks to MSG Nieto, WO Brown and the staff of super excellent cooks. He may be contacted at:

jimcampbell1st@hotmail.com.

THE CAMPBELL SCALE

During a counseling session with a very prominent businessman, he asked, "How am I doing?"

I said, "You are doing fine."

He said, "I know I am growing. I can feel it. However, knowing you, I know you have criteria somewhere in your mind that you use to make the determination about how well I am doing. I am a businessman. What I want to know is:

"Where was I, on a scale of 1 to 10, when I started?
Where am I now?
How far do I have to go?
How long will it take to get there?
What do I have to do to get there?
How much will it cost?"

I informed him I thought he was at about 2.8. He, believing he had been a 10.0 all his life, did not bat an eye. He simply asked, "What makes you say that?

I told him people go through 4 phases – Unawareness, New Conclusions, Growth, and Harmony. I said it takes about 30 hours to discover the Unawareness - or the X to N theory. It takes about a year of developing new beliefs to reach the Growth Mode. A person then moves gradually toward the 10.0 end of the scale for the rest of his or her life. I have never met anyone who is a 10.0!

This conversation prompted me to design the scale on the following page. I am hoping we can one day develop a measurement test to determine where a person falls within the scale. It would be nice even to distinguish between tenths of a point – e.g., 1.1 and 1.2.

CAMPBELL SCALE

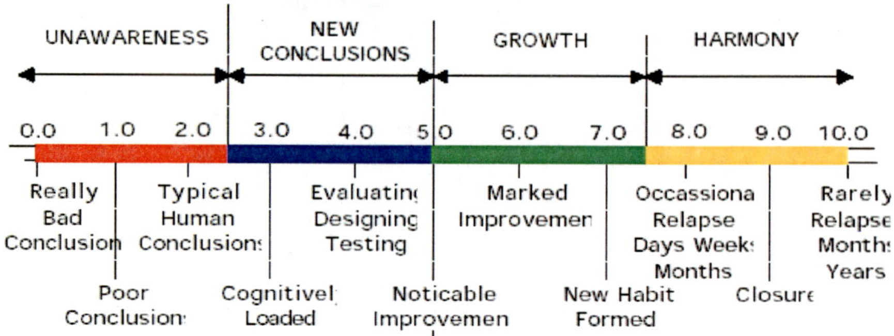

UNAWARENESS
Justifies behaviors
Rationalizes actions
Unawareness prevalent
Transient relationships
Emotionally isolated
Guilt over poor decisions
Harmful to self and others
Condition deteriorating
Life is painful
Tried everything - nothing works
Blames failure on others

MAKING NEW CONCLUSIONS
More open to feedback
Increased self awareness
Commited to learning more
Evaluating old conclusions
Designing new conclusions
Testing new conclusions
Excited by possibilities
Making new friends
Enjoys discussing change
Distinguish persons& patterns
Self condemnation ending

GROWTH
Significant closure on problems
Self Esteem more appropriate
Life direction established
New habits formed acceptably
Renewing of old relationships
Restoration of damages begins
No longer pushing others away
No guilt over past C B R
Accountable for personal behavior

HARMONY
Life goals being achieved
Equal Value - self & others
Controls time & attention
Involved in Culture progress
Turned outward not inward
Transmits personal security
Productive citizen
Experiencing the joy of life
Emotionally stabalized
Helping others become

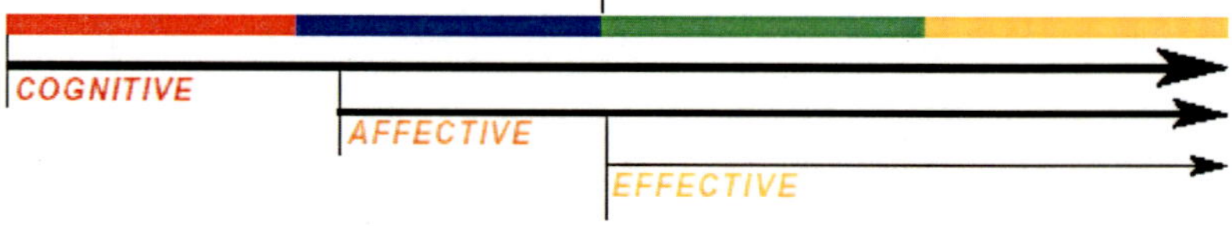

ORDER ◦ CONTINUITY ◦ CUMULATIVE

 "THECAMPBELLSCALE" PAGE1/1